NEUROLOGICAL BIRDSONG

NEUROLOGICAL BIRDSONG

A.J. LEES

MIRABEAU PRESS

Published by Mirabeau Press

PO Box 4281

West Palm Beach, FL 33401

ISBN: 978-1-7357055-6-9

First Edition

MIRABEAU

CONTENTS

FOREWORD

Every generation of doctors, once it has reached a certain stage of life, laments the loss of some aspect of past practice: and perhaps this is as it should be, for what a wretched life it must have been if there had been nothing in it whose loss would rightfully be regretted!

Andrew Lees, however, is no Luddite who wants an end to technology and scientific advance, so that everything should remain forever the same. He was himself one of the world's most eminent researchers into a terrible and cruel malady, Parkinson's Disease, and knows well the benefits that science can bring. But the loss of humanity in a profession supposedly devoted to the welfare of humanity, a loss that certain modern developments have wrought, is also a terrible and cruel thing, as many a patient can attest, as he is treated as but a nut or a bolt on an assembly line, or even as a spanner in the works. Patients do get in the way of administration so!

In these aphorisms, gleaned from a lifetime's clinical experience, Professor Lees lays bare the pathology of modern medicine and its underlying causes. This pathology is not unique to medicine, and when he says that he learned as much from teachers whom he wished not to imitate as from those whom he did wish to imitate, he is suggesting a general principle, that a bad example can be a good example where it is reflected upon in order to expunge any tendency to the same badness in oneself. Moreover, since human beings are imperfect and rarely all of a piece, a person who is bad in one respect may be good in another. In one simple aphorism, then, Lees calls us to the exercise of right judgment, that inescapable duty of us all.

Many times, I wanted to shout 'Hurrah!' while reading this brief book, for example when Lees excoriates electronic medical records which so often make a fetish of information-gathering for its own sake, a repetitious quasi-religious ceremony, a substitute for reflection on the meaning of the information gathered. He is against the kind of inhuman medicine in which patients are simply scanned (by what one physician in my hospital called 'the answering machine') but not listened to or even examined. This, of course, is not the same as decrying scanners *per se*: it is, rather, a call to humane judgment in their use.

Medical care is an important component of modern society, perhaps increasingly so, and it is in dialectical relationship to the rest of society. No profession is an island entire of itself. Therefore, while Professor Lees' aphorisms will be of particular interest to doctors, nurses and others involved in medical care (perhaps even to managers!), they have much to say to the general public.

Theodore Dalrymple

INTRODUCTION

I loved the immediacy of Twitter and the possibility it gave to subvert an unsuspecting audience. It was a new box to play in and had similarities to graffiti and subway poetry. In its halcyon days it made me feel as if I had joined an exclusive club, where casual exchanges of ideas around a water cooler had the potential to change the culture of the world. Twittering offered me the chance to interact on an equal footing with young people starting off in medicine and thousands of people living with chronic neurological disorders. I tried to crystallise my ideas and strongest feelings in a perfect tweet (twoosh) of exactly 140 characters, as if it were a haiku.

To my surprise, I started to receive compliments from younger colleagues at the hospital. Ibrahim Imam, a British neurologist and author of *Surfing the Brain*, then started to repost some of my tweets on his *Neurochecklists* platform and graciously offered to help collate them for this book. As a young doctor, I had kept a notebook in the pocket of my white coat and had written down anecdotes that my teachers imparted on ward rounds. I have digested their wisdom and regurgitated it here in the form of birdsong. In some cases, I have reformatted the bald prose of the original tweets into a more poetic form.

For those who are suffering with neurological disability, I hope that my distant calls from the treetops will offer comfort, however miniscule, and for those physicians who have become unhappy, I hope this book will offer them support and encouragement to continue to preserve and renew life through their skill and humanity.

A. J. Lees
The National Hospital, Queen Square, London

A. OBSERVATION

1.
Over the summer months,
I have been plotting the mysterious comings and goings
of the birds.
In this chaos,
the sunflower gives me
the stability and soulfulness I need.
"Ah Sunflower, weary of time,
Who countest the steps of the sun".

2.
John Clare[1] was a field worker.
A natural scientist who did not shoot, stuff, dissect,
or arrange specimens.
He did not measure,
or spend time meticulously classifying.
But he observed the living world in all its beauty.
I have tried to follow his example,
and apply his method to the clinic.

---

[1] John Clare (1793-1864) was an English poet and naturalist.

3.

Sometimes before the start of out-patient clinics,
I sit tucked away in a corner of the waiting room,
busying myself with paperwork,
but at the same time watching,
and observing.

4.

The obvious tends to be invisible,
until some fool draws attention to it.

5.

Watch the patient enter the room,
and walk towards the chair.
Look at her face,
her clothes,
and her jewellery.
Look at the nails and smell the breath.
None of this is possible with telemedicine.

B. Patients

6.

Patients are far more than a bundle of diagnoses.

7.

If allowed to speak freely without interruption,
people present their complaints
in an average of 7 minutes.
Further thoughtful open-ended questions are then needed.

8.

If someone tells you they are not feeling themselves,
leave no stone unturned.

9.

Can you believe
that some doctors think
the family history can be obtained
just by asking a patient to fill in a form?
People conceal and forget detail
even more than they do
when filling in income tax returns.
When chasing a hereditary cause,
never forget the two-source rule.

10.

A physician should not feel pressure
to declare everything she knows,
if she believes it is not in the patient's best interest.

C. Diagnosis

11.

I cannot understand how a healthy person without
symptoms can be told
that they have a disease
or even a syndrome.
Based on my current understanding of these medical
words,
this is misleading.

12.

A medical fact is an interpretation based on a reading.
It is made from data,
which may include scientific measurement.

13.

As I have got older,
I have got quicker at making a diagnosis.
But at the same time,
I need longer for the consultation,
and my carapace of objectivity is more easily breached.

14.

At the end of taking the medical history,
it is important to have a clear understanding
of the primary complaint,
its duration,
and how it began.
Simple stuff,
but not always straightforward.
It requires attentive listening and experience.

15.

Neurological diagnosis is extremely challenging.
It takes years of apprenticeship under grand masters,
it can only be learned in the clinic and the ward.
It is not a virtual subject,
practised in a virtual hospital.

16.

The medical history is complex data,
waiting for clinical interpretation.
Even a poem is a type of data.

17.

When I am faced with a clinical conundrum,
I first ask advice from a colleague.
If there is no answer,
I may seek a further opinion,
and if there is still no resolution,
I may refer on to a physician in another hospital.
Textbooks are of little use in this situation.

18.

You cannot reduce the clinical picture
to a series of scales and tick boxes,
administered by health care professionals
who have not been taught clinical skills during their
training.

19.

I am opposed to the notion,
favoured by many medical academics,
that a person can have a "non-harmful" diagnosis,
and a malady that does not cause suffering.
'Inconsequential disease'.
Not my kind of doctoring.

D. Education

20.

Concentrate on improving the art of history taking
at medical school. Students must present their findings to
their teachers and accept suggestions for improvement.

21.

Academic neurology departments
should reward outstanding teachers with promotion.

22.

A system that denies trainees
the opportunity to watch master clinicians taking a history,
and examining at the bedside,
is second rate.
As Osler[2] knew,
the lecture hall and the library
cannot substitute for learning on the job.

---

[2] William Osler (1849-1919) was a Canadian physician who was
one of the first doctors to pioneer 'hands on' bedside clinical
training. He is frequently described as the Father of Modern
Medicine.

23.

During my career in neurology,
I have learned as much,
if not more,
from those I do not resemble,
and have no wish to resemble,
as from those who seem more plausibly assigned to me
as role models.

24.

I learned how to decide if a patient was ill or not
in 20 minutes.
But it was quasi-veterinary and not without risk.
In those days we had far more beds to admit people.
Any ordered investigations should ideally
now be carried out on the same day.

25.

Electronic learning is always inferior
to the experience of listening
to an inspirational speaker
live and unplugged.

26.

For those on a wanderjahre,
you need to hitch up with a master
who sees patients in clinic,
does rounds,
and enjoys sharing wisdom.

27.

How to take a history:
Watch your mentor in clinic and at the bedside,
then throw yourself in the deep end and practice.
Practice on patients.
Interviews conducted by detectives on suspects
are very different.

28.

I find most neurology residents to be bright as buttons,
sharp as knives,
and keen to receive clinical instruction.
The problem stems from the increasing distance
between some departmental chairmen and the bedside,
and the fact that many place a very low priority
on education.

29.

I remember with affection the "happy givers"
in the Leeds Naturalists' Club[3],
my instructors at The London Hospital[4],
and my mentors in neurology,
who showed me what to do.
All of them involved me,
and helped me understand.

30.

In some universities,
medical students are taken to art galleries,
to improve powers of observation.
Next, they'll be tuning them in to Bach,
to improve listening.
Anything to avoid the hospital bedside
and talking to the sick.

---

[3] The Leeds Naturalists' Club and Scientific Association was
founded in 1870 and has maintained a close relationship with
Leeds University.
[4] The London Hospital (now the Royal London Hospital) in
Whitechapel was founded in 1740. Its college was the first medical
school in England and Wales to be organised in connection with a
hospital.

31.

Spend a stage overseas during your training.
Keep your own personal notes
of all the cases you see in clinic and on the wards.
Write down the aphorisms and anecdotes your teachers
impart.

32.

The core skills of good doctoring remain unchanged
but society and technology
are constantly evolving.

33.

With the exception of "El Hombre Invisible"[5]
and my father, a schoolmaster,
all my mentors have been doctors and nurses,
who have shown a kindly interest towards me.
Through their own tangible determination
to make poorly people better,
they have inspired me to try harder.

---

[5] In my book *Mentored by a Madman: The William Burroughs Experiment*
(Notting Hill Editions, 2016), I describe how the writer of *Naked
Lunch* became an invisible mentor during my training and then in
my clinical research. Burroughs was known in Tangier as 'El
Hombre Invisible' because he deliberately made himself as
insignificant and unobtrusive as possible.

E. Discovery

34.

To be an innovator,
one must risk making a fool of oneself,
and sometimes be prepared to admit error in public.

35.

3 groups have been steamrollered
by the big battalions and current dogma:
The maverick "Little Man",
The Princes of Serendip,
and The Researcher who observes
what everyone else has seen
but thinks what no one has thought before.

36.

Are you still curious,
to investigate the cause of symptoms,
and to find answers for patients' questions,
for which you have no answer?
Is this still possible as a clinical academic?

37.

It is intriguing to contemplate,
that the Nobel Prize in Physiology and Medicine,
has been given only twice,
for innovative treatment of nervous disorders.
In 1927 to Wagner-Jauregg for the use of malaria to treat
neurosyphilis.
And in 1949 to Egas Moniz for leucotomy.

38.

John Cade[6], the curious innovator,
and Mogens Schou[7], the man who never gave up,
saved thousands of creative people from committing
suicide.
Never let the lithium flame go out.

---

[6] John Frederick Joseph Cade (1912-1980) was an Australian
psychiatrist who in 1948 discovered the mood stabilising effects of
lithium in manic-depressive psychosis.
[7] Mogens Schou (1918-2006) was a Danish psychiatrist whose
research and championing of lithium eventually led to its use as the
treatment of choice for bipolar disorder.

39.

A gazpacho of serendipity, science,
and technological advance,
has led to so many medical discoveries.
But why is one of the ingredients
always written out of the experiment?
It is as if chance observation
diminishes the achievement.
Far from it!

40.

Leaders of our profession
often concede with gritted teeth,
that breakthroughs in medicine,
can come from the unlikeliest of people and places.
I would go further and say that they nearly always do,
in the treatment of brain disorders.

41.

Nothing is true;
everything is permitted.
Don't let your wild ideas or convictions
dissipate in a labyrinth.
Light a torch,
and keep exploring the darkness.

42.

Reward risk,
and sometimes what grant committees refer to
disparagingly
as fishing trips.
Dismantle the bureaucracy
that is stifling science.
Bring back self-experimentation,
and encourage citizen science.

43.

When one sets off to find the lost camel,
it is an advantage to include the arabesque,
and the content of dreams,
in your search for clues.

44.

When we were trying to get people
to believe in dopamine dysregulation[8],
I remembered Dr Gooddy's[9] words,
that he had learned from his own teacher Frances
Walshe[10],
about the three stages of medical discovery.
First, it's not true.
Second, it's not important.
And finally, it was known all the time.

---

[8] Dopamine dysregulation is a clinical syndrome caused by misuse
and overuse of L-DOPA by patients with Parkinson's disease.
[9] William Walton Gooddy (1916-2004) was an English neurologist.
He was one of my first chiefs at University College Hospital. He
took an interest in me and recommended I read the Sherlock
Holmes canon and Marcel Proust as an essential part of my clinical
apprenticeship.
[10] Sir Francis Rouse Walshe (1885-1973) was an eminent English
neurologist who held staff appointments at the National Hospital,
Queen Square and University College Hospital, London.

F. BURNOUT

45.

Another reason burnout is increasing,
is that it has become increasingly difficult for UK
neurologists
to build clinical research into their job plan.
The few gaps get filled by dreary administration,
mandatory training courses, committees filled with impotent
gloom, and private practice.

46.

Any neurologist who goes through the motions,
behaving like a government functionary,
or allows herself to be bullied,
or manipulated by health insurance companies,
will combust quickly.

47.

David Marsden[11] used to say that,
when he was feeling tired of committees,
or frustrated with academic bureaucracy,
he would look forward
to his clinic days at 8-11 Queen Square.
Surely this, a walk round the block and teaching,
are the best antidotes to academic burnout?

48.

Preventing burnout
will require a concerted unified effort,
to re-establish a culture
free from the commercial regulations and excessive
accountability
that have been imposed on doctors.

---

[11] Charles David Marsden (1938-1998) was an English neurologist and clinical neuroscientist who founded a school of neurology in his subspeciality of movement disorders. He worked at Kings College Hospital and later became the Dean of the Institute of Neurology, Queen Square where we were colleagues and friends.

49.

The solution to burnout,
is to re-establish the original motivations,
that led a physician
to pursue medicine in the first place.

50.

When I felt fed up at work,
I used to listen to a few tracks
from the Detroit Spinners[12],
and then go and see some patients
in Charles Symonds House[13].
Drinking cups of tea
in self-aggrandising gatherings,
and making polite chit chat to administrators,
was deadly tiring.

---

[12] The Detroit Spinners are an American rhythm and soul group who had their peak success in the 1970s with hits like 'Could it be I'm Falling in Love' and 'Working my Way Back to You'.
[13] Charles Symonds House, named after a distinguished English neurologist who worked at the National Hospital, was a building opposite the main hospital in Queen Square where neurology clinics were held on the ground floor.

51.
Soul music helped me better understand
the despair of loneliness,
the importance of love,
and the individuality of every person.
During the Covid epidemic it became a powerful healing
force
and an extracurricular form of instruction.

G. CLINICAL NEUROLOGY

52.

Neurology is endlessly fascinating.

53.

Knowledge is the neurologist's lodestar,
but should rarely be evident during the consultation.

54.

The medical history is part of the romance.
We must keep a patient's life close to our souls.
Science underpins modern medicine but healing is an art.

55.

Neurologists should enthuse
over the beauty of high-touch medicine,
and challenge payers
to reimburse it appropriately.

56.

"Romantic" is a term
of condescending defamation.
It is often now applied
to disparaging avant-garde positions.
It is a lost dimension I want to resurrect,
so that it becomes a subversive truth,
which disturbs the mechanical deterministic process.

57.

Neurologists who aspire
to become top notch basic scientists,
inevitably fall between two stools.
But clinical research is something
we should all be doing.

58.

Neurologists,
however specialised,
should never get cut off
from general medicine.
It is a cardinal error.

59.

Neurology is about making patterns,
as well as their recognition.
We make the blind see,
the lame walk.
A grain of gadolinium[14] can't do that.

60.

No place for mediocrity
in life or in neurology.

---

[14] Gadolinium is a paramagnetic chemical element with atomic number 64 that is used as a contrast agent for magnetic resonance imaging (MRI).

61.

Payers need to understand
that if the neurological consultation is rushed,
medical error is inevitable.

62.

Referred neurological symptoms
demand a face-to-face medical interview,
a focused examination,
and to be seen by a consultant.

63.

Residents learn bad habits from teachers
who believe neurology can be reduced to metrics.
These people only pay lip service to listening,
to observation,
and to inference
It is time for patients to stand up against this.

64.

The department[15] ran itself once I had settled in.
Everything depended on quality control,
the knack of sniffing out talent,
making the rising stars
feel they were part of an exclusive orchestra.
I was Hank Cosby[16],
blowing my horn occasionally in the background
of each new Motown symphony.

65.

The key to problem solving in neurology,
is not an overstuffed brain attic,
but an ability to perceive detail,
that others have ignored.

---

[15] The Reta Lila Weston Institute for Neurological Studies at
University College London where I was Director from 1998-2013.
[16] Henry R. Cosby (1928-2002) was a saxophonist, song writer and
arranger at Motown Records, Detroit. I tried to model my
department on Motown chairman Berry Gordy's business model: a
close-knit family, healthy competition, and a loving environment.

66.

The multiplicity of clinical presentations in neurology,
is why we still lay so much store
on the consultation.
But it is my experience,
that all good doctors
know its value.

67.

In my view,
the place for telemedicine,
is miniscule in neurology.
I don't want to practice what is second best
for political expediency or profit.

68.

The pleasure that comes,
from diagnosing a treatable disorder
that has been missed,
is the neurologist's nearest equivalent
to scoring a goal.
But it must be kept to oneself.
Humility is an English doctor's favourite form of vanity.

69.

There are symptoms that present to neurologists,
that we consistently misdiagnose,
or fail to label.
Referral to a different specialist,
leads to prompt denouement.
Is it that they did not feature in our textbooks,
and were not embraced by our teachers?

70.

There is a case for strength in numbers in neurology,
but only if the opportunity it provides,
is used to exchange ideas,
to share experiences which advance our field,
and result in tangible improvements in patient care.
Like Henry Ford[17],
I also believe competition breeds champions.

---

[17] Henry Ford (1863-1947) was an American industrialist and
business magnate who founded the Ford Motor Company and the
assembly line technique of mass production in Detroit, Michigan.

H. Soulful Neurology

71.

Our rational speciality needs romance and soul,
to take us to the next platform of discovery.

72.

Diagnosis is vital and is often not straightforward,
but it is the easiest part
when one is dealing with
chronic neurological impairment.
Managing change is much more challenging.

73.

The daily practice of neurology strengthens the mind
But it is by attending,
and in the art of healing,
that it becomes soulful,
as well as stimulating.

74.

Romantic science is an old
and rather denigrated term.
But my coinage of the term soulful neurology,
is a call to arms,
for psychiatrists and neurologists
who are interested in the lives of the people
who ask for their help.

75.

Soulful neurology embraces the subjective,
the qualitative
and the biographical.
The essence of a human being.

76.

Soulful neurology is characterised by
a wider imaginative dimension,
the magic that lurks beneath the infallible,
a sixth sense,
and altamirage[18].

---

[18] Altamirage is that special personal quality by which good luck is
prompted as a result of personally distinctive actions. It is a concept
that was developed by the neurologist and Zen master James H.
Austin, who spent time during his training at the National Hospital
with Macdonald Critchley.

77.

Soulful neurology is underpinned
by an immaculate clinical method
that involves silent listening,
astute noticing,
and abductive reasoning.

78.

Soulful neurology
values twentieth century scientific reductionism
in helping to localise the site of the lesion.
But wants to combine it
with the rich and complex tapestry of human behaviour
that existed in the nineteenth century.

79.

Try to give your right cerebral hemisphere
more than just a brief daily workout,
and neurology will become soulful
and dare I say,
fun.

I. Parkinson's Disease

80.

I've always tried the drugs I prescribe.
Levodopa made me terribly sick.
It wasn't anywhere near as nice as apomorphine.
But the best of all was selegiline -
being on a monoamine oxidase inhibitor for a week
was energising.

81.

Three areas of academic focus
I'd like to see less of
in Parkinson's disease:
New scales especially for non-motor symptoms,
Functional imaging where no attempt is made
to validate the findings by post mortem studies,
And division of PD into subtypes
based on Lewy body distribution.

82.

A feeling of trembling inside has many causes,
including anxiety and caffeine.
But it is very common in Parkinson's disease,
occurring in some people years before bradykinesia,
rigidity
or rest tremor.

83.

Alpha synuclein[19] accumulation in tissues is certainly a
clue,
but I have always been intrigued
by elderly people with Braak stage 6[20] Lewy body
pathology,
who had no symptoms or signs
of Parkinson's disease in life.

---

[19] Alpha synuclein is a nerve cell protein that regulates the release
of neurotransmitters at the synapse. An aggregation of misfolded
alpha synuclein is commonly found in the brains of people with
Parkinson's disease.
[20] Braak's method of staging described in 2003 is based on a
hypothesis that alpha synuclein aggregation begins in the
peripheral tissues and then spreads into the central nervous system.
Stage 6 is the most severe stage and signifies that the disease has
invaded several regions in the cerebral cortex.

84.

Cotzias[21] was the first to state in 1969
that it was impossible to determine the therapeutic
response
of an individual patient
without a trial of DOPA,
that "intermittencies" in response occurred early,
and that tolerance was not seen.
It was not Mel Yahr[22] as often stated.
Putting the record straight.

85.

I filled in the Non-Motor Symptoms Questionnaire
for Parkinson's disease,
and ticked 10 out of 30 boxes.
I see no advantage to dishing this pseudo-metric out
to people with Parkinson's disease
before, or on arrival at the clinic.

---

[21] George Cotzias (1918-1977) was a Greek clinical scientist who in
1967, while working at the Brookhaven National Laboratory in the
USA, was the first to convince the world that L-DOPA was an
efficacious treatment for Parkinson's disease.
[22] Melvyn Yahr (1917-2004) was Houston Merritt Professor of
Neurology at Columbia University College of Physicians and
Surgeons in New York and a leading figure in the early studies on
L-DOPA in Parkinson's disease.

86.

I have always been much more interested
in identifying the smaller number of patients
with Parkinson's disease
who will benefit from a particular treatment,
than the far larger number,
who might.

87.

I saw a patient with early Parkinson's disease
whose first symptom
was an inability to spread butter evenly
over his morning toast.
After all these years,
I am still collecting and fascinated by,
new clinical presentations.

88.

I still look at people with Parkinson's disease
with a sense of wonderment,
and a feeling
that I have barely scratched the surface,
of a chaotic condition.
If I can acquire different ways of seeing,
then I will hopefully gain
important new vistas of understanding.

89.

I'm looking for other people with Parkinson's disease,
who find dancing releases the shackles.
The 1977 Dancing Queen,
at Talk of the North Cleethorpes Pier all-nighters
can't have been a one-off?

90.

Most patients with Parkinson's disease
have no complaints of loss of sense of smell
at the time of diagnosis.
No REM sleep behaviour disorder.
No constipation.
No tremor.
And no late onset depression.
Like so much else,
the prodrome is being inflated,
and this will lead to error and bogus concepts.

91.

Long ago I started to ask
about oneiric content
in people with Parkinson's disease.
I have three looking glass dreamers
in whom recurrent nightmares
involved time space slowing up,
several who found tricks against freezing in dreams
and one who imagined they could run and move normally
while asleep.

92.

Neurologists raise eyebrows
when I tell them that championing apomorphine
has been my greatest achievement.
I hope it will be resurrected too,
for the control of acute craving in alcoholism.

93.

The overall incidence of Parkinson's disease
is probably not increasing,
despite all the 'epidemic' hype.

94.

Nobody ever thought Parkinson's disease
was an "old person's disease",
unless you call early 60s,
its peak age of onset,
old.
The incidence seems to actually decline
in the tenth decade of life.

95.

Ordering a Parkinson gene panel,
and then being informed the patient has a rare mutation,
is pleasing.
But unlike accurate clinical diagnosis
the sensation is momentary.

96.

Some neurologists desire
to spend less contact time with the patient
through the use of pre-visit questionnaires.
But if used effectively as an aide-memoire by the patient,
and gone over thoughtfully by the doctor,
it should extend the consultation time.

97.

The differences in the treatment of Parkinson's disease,
are greater now than in 1965.
A drug may give clinically meaningful improvement,
but still not be offered.
National opinion leaders and patient influencers,
are two reasons for the remarkable variations in
prescribing.

98.

The mere presence of aggregated alpha synuclein in a
tissue or organ,
does not mean that the structure is sick,
or diseased.
One in ten healthy elderly people have Lewy bodies[23] in
the brain.

---

[23] Lewy bodies are bullseye inclusions that develop inside nerve
cells and contain alpha synuclein protein.

99.

To test bradykinesia[24],
I ask the patient to tap each finger against the thumb
for 20 seconds.
I also ask for fast bilateral hand movements,
Imitating 'mouth of crocodile opening and closing'.
Not the UPDRS[25] way.
Activating methods are also sometimes necessary.

100.

Three pieces of existing dogma in Parkinson's disease
that I hope will be challenged more:
That its prevalence
has doubled in thirty years.
That amnesia is an integral part
of the primary disease process.
That Lewy bodies spread
from the periphery to the brain.

---

[24] Bradykinesia is a *sine qua non* for the diagnosis of Parkinson's disease characterised by a progressive reduction in speed and amplitude on finger tapping.
[25] The Unified Parkinson's Disease Rating Scale (UPDRS) is a commonly used clinical measurement to follow the course of Parkinson's disease.

101.

I understand that the EMA[26] and the FDA[27]
insist on benefit over placebo
in evaluating efficacy.
But I tell my patients
that device assisted therapies
improve "daily on-time" in Parkinson's disease
by 4 or more hours,
not the 2 hours
quoted in the trial publications.

102.

You can't reduce Parkinson's disease,
to a series of measurements,
especially if they are of questionable biological
significance.
The most informative staging of PD
depends only on the age of the patient,
and the duration of disease.

---

[26] EMA is the European Medicines Agency.
[27] FDA is the United States Food and Drug Administration.

J. GOOD MANNERS

103.

I dislike uninvited, assumed informality.

104.

My advice for old neurologists:
Don't bore your colleagues with anecdotes
about an imaginary golden age.
Instead tell them about your worst mistakes.
Curb your growing brashness in meetings.
Don't try to start all over,
or envy youth.

105.

My advice for young neurologists:
Never follow the money.
The neurological literature began
before the new millennium.
Modesty and decency are still qualities
to be cultivated.

106.

Sometimes it seems to me as if the word *placebo*,
like the words *in my experience*,
should not be used in polite medical society.

107.

As a junior I called my chiefs "sir",
like "monsieur" in French.
It was not 'brown-nosing'
but a mark of my respect.
I was pleased to learn,
that at least in surgical specialities,
patients are still often referred to
as "sir" and "madam".

K. Elevated Practice

108.
"Doing nothing",
as it is offensively referred to by payers,
is often priceless.
It should be charged at a level
that reflects its value to the patient.

109.
A doctor should try in his daily work,
to make the conditions of human life more bearable,
by the alleviation of suffering,
and not continually strive to prolong survival at any cost.

110.
A neurologist should have wide-ranging curiosity and
inventiveness,
and an eagerness to discover something new.

111.

Doctors deal in nuance,
and the best know the right words to use,
for the right patient,
at the right time.
And when to stay silent.

112.

All my career I have been aware
of the privilege and responsibility
that being a doctor brings.
But I cannot do my best
in a sterile target-driven ambience,
where every last bit of fun
has been rubbed out by the system.

113.

I want to feel the desire to 'take one for the team',
not clock off at 5 pm.

114.
Always guard against wilful myopia.

115.
Any doctor who says to a patient,
"I know how you feel",
needs retraining.
Compassion is what is needed,
but it takes courage and kindness,
and unlike empathy cannot be taught.

116.
Being competent and kind,
and trying to relieve suffering,
is what doctors strive to achieve.
But they should also try to find answers,
for the questions that their patients ask and
which they cannot answer.
This involves curiosity,
and needs dedicated time.

117.

Double check your sources and
be a light unto yourself.

118.

Do what you know is right,
not what you are told you can do.
Never be fobbed off.

119.

Don't let all those theories,
and systematic classifications,
clutter your brain.
Don't be satisfied with what is known,
and what you are told you can prescribe.
Unfettered, unbiased observations
are what drive medicine forward.

120.

For those physicians,
who like the sound of their own voice,
or suffer from "The Yacks",
always remember that "the Word is a Virus".
There is immense value
in brief golden silences during the consultation.

121.

Go that extra step for your patient,
even if it means challenging the committees.

122.

Hope, love and faith:
Healing forces that all the best physicians unconsciously
possess.

123.

How I missed my white coat
when they were banned.
Wearing it demanded a commitment
to science and purity,
and a weekly visit to the laundry.

124.

Professors, professors how often do you invite someone,
from an entirely different faculty,
to give a talk in your department?

125.

How often do scientific programme committees consider
inviting a historian,
a sociologist,
a novelist,
a mathematician,
or even an anthropologist,
to give a keynote lecture
at a neurology conference?

126.
I am always looking
for differences among the working men and women
in the crowd.
Little details that distinguish them,
one from another
in the battle of life.

127.
I believe and trust in people who,
through long experience
and making mistakes,
have improved their performance, precision,
and competence.

128.
I have never prescribed a tune for a patient,
but on rare occasions,
when my own words have felt entirely inadequate,
I have recommended a poem.

129.

I like my scientists to be modest,
hesitant, and sceptical.
And to have an old school gentility.

130.

I miss the saturnine, cultured mavericks,
who inspired me to light candles,
and stop cursing the darkness.
I miss the rough and tumble debates,
where we were all devil's advocates.

131.

I prefer to use my limited time,
in a follow-up consultation,
searching for hidden agendas.
These are far beyond the scope
of any quality-of-life checklist.

132.

I still get lasting satisfaction
from localising a lesion
by neurological examination.
I still enjoy hearing a clinical presentation
I have never encountered before.

133.

I try to pick up on the casual asides
during a consultation.
They help me understand what makes patients tick,
and why they are able to go on.

134.

I used to bring patients into hospital,
solely for medical observation,
which sometimes led to the diagnosis.

135.

I want my doctor to act
with enormous self-confidence,
to be cheering and reassuring,
to heal me not only with her expertise,
but by the fact that disease or anxiety,
are incompatible with her welcome presence.

136.

I want to look into my doctor's eyes,
and watch his or her expression,
when I have a medical problem.

137.

I'm all for the alleviation of suffering through listening,
but unlike Ivan Illich[28], author of Medical Nemesis,
I'm also a fan of science.

---

[28] Ivan Illich (1926-2002) was a Roman Catholic priest,
philosopher and social critic who argued that modern medicine
had damaged human health by disease mongering and iatrogenic
harm.

138.

If you prescribe no medication,
you may be doing your patient no harm.
But if you are able to make them laugh,
you may be doing them a lot of good.

139.

If you stay on Twitter now it is X,
beware of recommender algorithms,
and irresponsible soundbites.

140.

In medicine and in life,
I question my actions every day.

141.

It has never surprised me,
that physiotherapists commonly
make the diagnosis of Parkinson's syndrome.
They see through their touch,
and never skimp the physical examination.

142.

It is not impossible
to combine the art of healing
with modern medicine.
Good doctors do it every day all over the world.

143.

My heroes are on the frontline,
showing kindness and compassion,
tapping reflexes,
wiping bottoms,
bringing comfort to all those in need.

144.

Never write a prescription
as if you were a postman
delivering a brown envelope.
Reassure the patient
that the risks of doing nothing
are greater than taking the medicine.

145.

Patients must be informed
about the common side effects of a treatment.
But this must always be counterbalanced
by an explanation of what benefits to expect.

146.

Personalised medicine
has been there from the start.
It was diminished
when vested interests hijacked EBM[29],
and guidelines stopped doctors thinking for themselves.
No clinician can be imprecise.

147.

Question everything,
dissent,
and if necessary fight back.
No blind obedience.
No e-patients[30].
No life-threatening rules.
Do what you know is right.

---

[29] Evidence Based Medicine

[30] An e-patient is a health consumer who participates fully in
his/her medical care, primarily by gathering information about
medical conditions that impact them and their families, using the
Internet and other digital tools.

148.
Truthful kindness is an unquantifiable remedy.
You can't put a price on that.

149.
Two elements of kindness are threatened,
by cutbacks and top down robotics.
The reduction of patient anxiety by timely care,
and the discretionary effort where a doctor goes the extra
step,
and exceeds patient expectation.
Both are invaluable healers.

150.
When I feel poorly I seek out a physician
who is genial, likeable,
and explains things clearly.
A mentalist.
Not a businessman,
or a scientist.

151.

When I'm staring down the barrel of my latest mistake,
I gather up the horror of it,
understand why,
accept it,
and realise there is something precious there,
from which I can learn for tomorrow.

152.

As far as clinical medicine is concerned,
I refuse to regard anecdotal evidence as lowly.
It is easy to learn the few Level 1 guidelines,
but to acquire clinical judgement and act on uncertainty,
requires common sense, experience,
and a love of people.

153.

As I slowly lost my grip
on the medical literature,
I gradually gained the courage
to listen to my patients more attentively.
I became more and more curious
about their lives.
I was no longer top dog,
but I was in greater demand than ever before.

154.
I have always been interested
in understanding the thinking and effort
that went into a method
that is now taken for granted in neurology.
The magic of semiotics, the physical examination
and the pathognomonic signs of disease.

L. THE OLD MASTERS

155.

Gordon Holmes[31] believed each neurological
examination,
should be as rigorous as a scientific experiment.

156.

"Je ne suis qu'un visuel",
Charcot[32] told Freud.
His method was practising nosography
but one could also call it botanising.
In the early days
he wanted to identify, classify
and describe nervous disease,
but then when he had created his museum of clinical facts,
he wanted to treat it too.

---

[31] Gordon Morgan Holmes (1876-1965) was an Anglo-Irish
neurologist who was on the staff at the National Hospital, Queen
Square and Charing Cross Hospital in London. He introduced the
painstaking physical examination of the nervous system which is
still used today.
[32] Jean-Martin Charcot (1825-1893) was a French physician who
worked at L'Hopital Salpetrière and is widely regarded as the
founder of neurology.

157.

Gowers[33] wrote thoughtfully about hysteria,
as did David Marsden.
Many of the early Queen Square staff,
like Risien Russell[34],
depended on cases of neurasthenia, hysteria and anxiety
to make a living.

158.

John Walshe[35] was a man of medical science
with immense integrity
and absolute dedication to his patients.
His refusal to play the game for political expediency
was what I admired most in him.

---

[33] William Gowers (1845-1915) was arguably the greatest clinical neurologist of all time and worked at University College Hospital and the National Hospital, Queen Square.
[34] James Risien Russell (1863-1939) was born in Demerara, Guyana and was on the staff of the National Hospital, Queen Square for 30 years. He had a large, exclusive private practice.
[35] John Michael Walshe (1920-2022), son of the neurologist Francis Walshe, was a clinical academic at Addenbrooke's Hospital, Cambridge who discovered two efficacious treatments for Wilson's disease, a hitherto fatal genetic disorder. After his retirement he returned to University College Hospital and the Middlesex Hospital where we did a Wilson's disease clinic together.

159.

No webinar will ever stick in my head,
like the first patient I saw with Parkinson's disease,
or a riveting Marsden or Stern[36] talk.

160.

How many chairmen of neurology departments,
talk about the writings of Miller Fisher,
Ray Adams,
Lou Caplan,
Bill Landau,
and the cardiologist Bernard Lown?
How many still do rounds?

---

[36] Gerald Malcolm Stern (1930-2018) was a Consultant
Neurologist at University College Hospital, London and an
international authority on Parkinson's disease. He was my mentor
and senior colleague and a charismatic teacher and orator.

161.

When presenting a patient to the class,
always begin by setting the scene.
Gowers did this in his lectures to the students at UCL,
and Harry Lee Parker[37] was another master at this.
In this way,
the presentation becomes more than a set of facts,
but a clinical picture.

162.

Charcot's eye saw what his mind did not yet know.
He understood that the difference
between adequate and inadequate observation,
and between looking and seeing,
was more than just a difference in degree.
It was absolute in its enduring influence.

---

[37] Harry Lee Parker (1894-1959) was an Irish and American
neurologist who worked at the Mayo Clinic. His book *Clinical
Studies in Neurology,* published in 1956, is an almost forgotten classic.

M. DIGITAL MEDICINE

163.

The advances of high-tech modern medicine
are simply astonishing to me.
But I regret that this has led to a very mechanical
approach
to patient management.

164.

Down with electronic health records.
How could we all be conned,
leading to the current catastrophe
of increasing medical misdiagnosis,
and neurologist burnout.

165.

Electronic health records are a form of totalitarianism,
which take away our professionalism,
and lead to second rate care.

166.
Electronic health records take you away
from being with the living breathing human being,
who has come to see you because she is ill.

167.
Frankly I would think that
people with cognitive impairment
are the least suitable of all groups
for telehealth.
Alzheimer's disease should never be
a diagnosis given remotely.
For those with cognitive impairment,
touch is vital,
and technology can be disorientating.

168.
High performance digital medicine.
I see it as a dehumanising force.
How about bringing an amanuensis back,
to prevent electronic systems
damaging the consultation?

169.

I am interpreting it as a legacy of Zoom,
where my colleagues are all now disembodied, talking
heads.
A technology that has diminished me to a voyeur,
and now haunts my dreams.

170.

I am talking here about internet consultations
leading up to diagnosis.
Seeing a domestic background
is not a domiciliary visit.
Online silences and a patient's voice are very different
from those appreciated in the consulting room.

171.

The host of variables in communication,
including the finely tuned silent tonalities
of body language,
mean that Artificial Intelligence
will never achieve healing,
even if it assists diagnosis.

172.

I have hardened my view about teleconsultation
used for patients with new neurological symptoms.
It is not better than nothing,
and it is medicolegally indefensible.
Doctors who succumb to it,
or accede to it,
should question if they are in the right job.

173.

If there is bad news or treatment options,
I want my doctor there in front of me
face-to-face.

174.

If we can restore rational, collective political action,
and rehabilitate thoughtful decision making,
it will be much easier to prevent Artificial Intelligence
becoming an unbroachable magic power.

175.

In medicine as in every walk of life,
technology is never neutral.
It cannot be isolated from the use to which it is put.

176.

Neurologists should avoid
"lowtouch hi-tech" clinical practice.
They also need to be skilful change advisors.

177.

Some claim that a video consultation
is OK for a first specialist consultation.
That it offers a window into a patient's home
akin to a domiciliary visit.
And that it is an upgrade
on a telephone consultation.
I question all three.

178.

Spending more and more time
grappling with electronic health records,
diminishes the joy of being a clinician.

179.

Telehealth,
including self-monitoring
with wearables and ingestible sensors,
is leading to remarkable changes in medicine.
But its ramifications,
with regard to quality of care,
and healing,
have received scant attention by its advocates.

180.

An efficient personal assistant with social skills, empathy,
and a healing telephone voice,
is what physicians need.
Not a half-baked electronic record system,
and a battalion
of impotent administrators.

N. Health Screening

181.

Selling sickness is now at an all-time high.
Exploiting patient's fears through the marketing of disease,
is a very profitable business.

182.

I would never have an **MRI** head screen.
I would never have a Carotid doppler check[38].
I would never have an ApoE4[39] test,
or a tau and amyloid[40] scan.
For now, if I remain asymptomatic,
I'd just like a face-to-face chat
with a wise and kindly practitioner.

---

[38] Carotid doppler screening is an ultrasound examination on the neck to check the circulation in the large blood vessels to the brain.
[39] ApoE4 is the most prevalent genetic risk factor for Alzheimer's disease and is offered by genomics and biotechnology companies like 23 and Me on the internet.
[40] Tau and amyloid are two proteins that when they aggregate into clumps in the brain are believed to be causative agents for Alzheimer's disease. Both can now be tested for using brain scans, lumbar punctures and blood tests.

183.

I have found telling patients the good news,
that an abnormal test requested by someone else,
is likely of no clinical significance,
as difficult as conveying bad news.
There are still very few diseases worth screening for.

184.

I try to be abstemious,
walk for an hour,
and keep an eye on my blood pressure.
But I cannot see how looking at MRI pictures,
of my clapped-out brain,
could give me hope.
It would make me anxious.
It's bad enough charting the senile blemishes,
mushrooming on my torso.

185.

I'm dead against the pursuit of health
as a pathway to surrogate salvation.

186.

I'm opposed to
meddlesome anticipatory medicine.

187.

The private sector testers make claims,
that more information is always better.
They provide no proof for this,
and brush off the disadvantages.

O. BAD SCIENCE

188.

It's the immodesty and certainty,
that has crept into modern science,
that concerns me.

189.

A study of 101 basic science discoveries
published in major journals,
and claiming a clinical application,
found that 20 years later,
only one had produced clinical benefit[41].
The corruption of Big Science,
is as bad as the corruption of clinical practitioners.

---

[41] This was a study published in 2003 by John Ioannides who
together with his wife examined 101 basic science discoveries
published in leading scientific journals such as *Nature* and *Cell*
between 1979 and 1983, all of which claimed to have a clinical
application. Twenty years on, only 27 of these technologies had
been tested clinically, five approved for marketing and only one
deemed to have clinical benefit.

190.

I dislike the ever-increasing number of scientists,
who are expansionists, opportunists,
and mislead the public for profit,
or for cynical self-advancement.

191.

Another holy cow in Parkinson's disease
is the neuroanatomical study of Braak.
Never replicated.
And without clinico-pathological correlations.

192.

What I crave is a return to that era
of infectious excitement and spontaneity,
where experimentation was driven by clinical curiosity,
and carried out by tight knit teams.
Not consortia.
Not patient partners.
Not cohorts.
You may be thinking bad or pseudoscience,
and you may be right.

193.

There seem to be more and more academic physicians
who dislike diagnosing and treating patients,
and would rather leave patient care to colleagues.
This is a big change from 25 years ago,
when many of the best clinicians were professors.

194.

Medical science
is far more than another flawed narrative.
In common with the rest of us,
scientists are subject to bias,
ambition and greed.
Their narrow reality
should never subvert proper doctoring.

195.

I reviewed a textbook on Alzheimer's disease,
with multiple references to the author's research,
but there was a complete absence of patients.
Not a single meaningful case history.
No sense of the impact dementia can have on a life.
Just self-promotion of guild science.

196.
"Aggressive diagnosis without net benefit",
is when a physician tells a patient
with a mini mental score of 28[42],
and abnormal tau and amyloid scans,
whose family are worried about "senior moments",
that she has Alzheimer's disease.

---

[42] The Mini Mental State Examination is a brief, commonly used set of questions for screening for cognitive impairment. The top score is 30 out of 30.

P. BAD MEDICINE

197.
Another ugly prefix has entered
the academic vernacular:
deep medicine,
deep phenotyping,
and deep learning.

198.
Deep medicine,
in common with precision,
personalised,
evidence-based
and narrative medicine,
demeans and deceives.
Those who use these terms
should read Osler and Gowers.

199.
Down with deep medicine.
Viva Bernard Lown[43].

200.
Down with impersonal no touch industrialised medicine.
Down with systems centred medicine.

201.
Eyes glued to the computer screen,
minutes wasted loading up scan images,
unnecessary scales and phone interruptions,
then giving a doleful prognosis in an attempt to be honest:
all powerful nocebos.

---

[43] Bernard Lown (1921-2021) was a Lithuanian-American
cardiologist who developed the direct current defibrillator for
cardiac resuscitation and introduced lidocaine for cardiac rhythm
disturbances. His autobiographical book *The Lost Art of Healing*,
published in 1996, describes how medicine in the United States of
America has strayed from its mission. In the book he writes,
'Words are the most powerful tool a doctor possesses, but words
like a two-edged sword can maim as well as heal'.

202.

I never found out who scrapped medical firms[44],

and allowed "safari"[45] ward rounds,

even in my own little hospital.

Try to heal, not just treat.

203.

The firm system,

at least in neurology,

was infinitely better

than the current chaos.

It was an educational and support system

for physicians.

---

[44] The medical firm system in hospitals was a model of medical apprenticeship where groups of doctors worked together to provide patient care. Firms generally had at least one permanent member, a consultant who led the firm and after whom it was named.

[45] Safari round is a disparaging term that has been given to physician- or surgeon-led ward rounds where the patients are scattered throughout the hospital in outlying wards rather than on a single ward as used to be the case in the past.

204.

Expensive technology and bogus measurements
lead to disease-mongering,
prediabetes, metabolic syndrome,
and now Alzheimer's disease.
Millions of consumers being frightened and mislead for
profit.

205.

But who is responsible
for rushing the hospital doctor?
Why does he or she have only ten minutes per patient?
What would be the repercussion,
if the clinic consultation lasted 30 minutes?
Reduced income?
Dismissal?

206.

I distrust citizen journalists who fanfare opinions,
who never bother to cross check their information,
who constantly denigrate experts,
and spread fear.

207.

I don't want to be told
that a patient is Yahr 3[46], UPDRS 22[47], MMS 20[48].
A litany of non-motor and quality of life scales,
attempting to describe a life in numbers.
For research, yes.
In the clinic, no.

208.

I think telehealth has brought into sharper focus,
the tension between vocation and business.
In the USA
medicine is an industry
controlled by health insurers and hospital administrators.

209.

In the wrong hands,
even the marvellous MRI head scan,
becomes a weapon.

---

[46] The Hoehn and Yahr scale is a commonly used system for
measuring disease progression in Parkinson's disease.
[47] Unified Parkinson's Disease Rating Scale
[48] Mini Mental Score

210.

Is it time to nationalise the pharmaceutical industry?
I am strongly in favour of the yes argument.
For Parkinson's disease,
where our very best drugs have been generic for decades,
there is a grave risk of them disappearing.

211.

Most healthy elderly people,
do not want to know,
that they have twice the risk of an incurable disease.
Coping with aging is hard enough.

212.

One thing that has got worse in hospital medicine,
is that physicians have been forced to be less interested in
their patients because of perceived boundaries and risk
aversion.

213.

Profit-driven motives,
insurance reimbursement schemes,
and outcome metrics.
These have transformed the landscape of medicine,
and estranged physicians from themselves,
and from their calling.

214.

Some reasons for "waste"
are tests ordered before patient examination,
screens not supported by good evidence,
repeated examinations at too short intervals,
and duplicate ordering with second opinions.

215.

Surely buzzers are not in use in hospital clinics?
If they are then I propose an immediate ban.

216.

The external reason leading to imaging "waste"
that I find most concerning,
is when a scan is ordered,
because of a doctor's intolerance
of diagnostic uncertainty.

217.

The medicine of previous years
had been based on the effort to single out important
syndromes,
by describing significant symptoms.
With the advent of the new instrumentation,
these classical forms of medical procedure
are being pushed into the background.

218.

The pre-visit questionnaire epidemic
is a sign of a disease called personal medical disinterest.
The "person of the patient" is less and less relevant.

219.

The appraisal system,
with continuing professional development diaries,
is a time consuming, self-reporting farce.
It fails in its aim
of protecting patients from bad and ignorant doctors.

220.

We are all storytelling animals
and should never be reduced to a bundle of nerves.

221.

We need to stop hiding behind bullshit protocols,
fake edicts,
and fear of sanction.
Get back to professionalism and sound clinical judgement.
Some patients take 2 minutes to sort out,
others more than an hour.

222.

Why is it that kindly doctors,
who fail to diagnose,
are punished and abused,
while those who cause unnecessary suffering,
from over-investigation and disease mongering,
are not?

223.

I sat on the front row
of the vast theatres,
packed with doctors
during the latest silly season of jamborees.
And as I listened to the keynote lectures,
I found myself asking the question:
"Are you for real?"
Impostors and Ted-talkers
had taken over the stage.

224.

Hyposkilliacs:
protocol-driven, unengaged,
condescending poor listeners,
who are not even pseudo-empathic.
They love flipping through notes,
interrupting,
ordering tests,
and proposing further referrals.
You can spot them
as soon as you walk in to the room.

Q. Bad Management

225.

Attempts to turn the beds of the National Hospital, Queen
Square
into a mere annexe of the adjoining laboratories
have so far failed.
But the threat of translocation is always there.

226.

All health care systems are failing,
partly because of Sisyphus syndrome,
and because of attempts to turn medicine
into a consumer driven market.
A physician now has to learn
how to subvert the system
both to survive,
and to maintain his professionalism and calling.

227.

Doctors have been infantilised,
unsupported,
and treated like untrustworthy delinquents
for the last 20 years.
It comes from the very top.
I favour a return
to the Medical Executive committee.
Most doctors who join management
become apparatchiks.

228.

Embracing and learning from error
is valuable for the basic scientist,
but the pernicious effect
of service bureaucracies and regulators on good doctors,
is harder to correct.
The truth is we are all now considered potential criminals.

229.

Medical scientists understand
the need for an open mind,
but they are forced to operate
within a gated community
which shuts out the curious bystander,
the hospital noticers,
and all the ordinary botanisers on the pavements.

230.

My heroes do not scuttle between offices,
attending meetings and laying down diktats,
creating distractions from the truth.

231.

The problem with targets
is that they measure what can be counted,
not what matters.
One less death and a hundred more patients,
crying out to be heard.

232.

We need to continue the fight
to preserve our vocation and professionalism
against those who wish to reduce medicine
to a technological business.

233.

When the CEO[49],
of a large not-for-profit US healthcare system,
builds himself a $14m home,
something is wrong with the system.

234.

Why did we all give in to the political gimmick,
that doctors must discard
their freshly laundered white coats?
It was an edict to reduce our respect,
and conceal the overcrowding and shortage
of isolation facilities in our hospitals.
I wore mine with pride.

---

[49] CEO is the acronym for Chief Executive Officer.

235.

I worry about universities
where teachers fear their own students,
and administrators strut about
like robber-barons.
Institutions where the next new signing
is all that matters
and where camaraderie
has been replaced by impact.

R. HOSPITALS

236.
A hospital's atmosphere
markedly influences
the healing process.

237.
Hospitals are like coral reefs.
They need nurturing and protecting.
Each one over many years
develops a distinctive microcosm
created by its organisms.

238.

When I arrived at the National Hospital[50],
I immediately felt at home.
The Victorian dimensions were human.
It had a feel, an atmosphere,
that suggested it was full of people,
acting responsibly and decently
who were trying to do well
by those they were concerned with.
I still get that feeling.

---

[50] Queen Square is the name, sometimes used by those who work there, for the National Hospital for Neurology and Neurosurgery in Bloomsbury, the historical cradle of British neurology.

S. RESEARCH

239.

The research I love has nothing to do with public health.
It stems from the patient.

240.

Forging research collaborations is impossible on Zoom.

241.

I greatly enjoyed sparring with Adrian Wills[51],
neurologist, author and aspirant boxing referee.
Bobbing and weaving are useful qualities for clinical
research,
so we were both in our element.

---

[51] Adrian Wills is a neurologist who is employed by Nottingham
University Hospitals NHS Trust.

242.

I had the good fortune to be there,
at the inception of agonists[52], MAOIB[53], Apomorphine[54]
and much later COMTI[55] in Parkinson's.
Everything we tested turned to gold,
and 3 times quicker than now.
A change in the process is needed.

243.

I remembered this morning a quote
that the late Maurice Pappworth[56] was very fond
of telling us at Seymour Hall Baths.
He likened statistics to bikinis,
in that they concealed what was vital,
while revealing much
that was occasionally interesting.

---

[52] Agonists is an abbreviation for dopamine agonist drugs.
[53] MAOIB is an acronym for Type B monoamine oxidase inhibitors.
[54] Apomorphine is a dopamine analogue.
[55] COMTI is an acronym for catechol-O-methyl-transferase inhibitors.
[56] Maurice Pappworth (1910-1994) was a charismatic medical tutor, physician and whistle-blower who ran renegade courses for junior doctors to help them pass the Royal College of Physicians examinations.

244.

I was a determined dilettante,
given a golden opportunity,
an unfettered tyro fishing in a mill pond after school,
with a string and a bent pin,
who, against all the odds,
hooked a monster.
Few heads of department then and no fat controllers.

245.

Most of my very best research was done
while I was a consultant at a teaching hospital.
I had no formal academic sessions,
but there was flexibility in the system
that allowed for free exchange,
between the university and the hospital.

246.

Much good work is being done in Parkinson's disease.
But more could be achieved,
if regulatory road blocks for clinical research were
lessened,
and the maverick was allowed a seat at the table.
Putting fortunes into one fashionable scientific bag,
has become a repetitive error.

247.

The science I fell in love with,
had honesty, disinterestedness and integrity,
and was without economic payoff.
How much of the "bullshit" overhyped research,
that underpins the current medical-industrial consortium,
fulfils this ideal?

248.

The ability to search the world literature
at the click of a mouse,
combined by our physiological need to forget,
puts us at severe risk of a retrograde amnesia,
for all literature more than 10 years old.
Beware people!

249.

I hope more funding will be made available,
for n=1 research[57] in Parkinson's disease,
in hospital and out in the real world.
Even n=10 clinical research projects,
would on some occasions be a step in the right direction.

---

[57] N=1 research is a clinical trial in which a single person
participates or one in which the investigator carries out self-
experimentation.

T. SCIENTIFIC PUBLISHING

250.

Being the senior author on a paper or an editor
is reminiscent of a butcher's trade.
It takes finesse and craftsmanship
to return the bloody corpse to a colleague
who has done all the hard graft.
Yet it is a necessary and valuable process.

251.

Dr Gooddy's advice:
"If it hasn't been written up in the last ten years,
write it up again
especially in a North American journal –
no one will remember".
The real lesson from this sad truth,
for those in training,
is to read
and quote the old literature when appropriate.

252.

I just learned that
some journals publish scientific papers online,
before the proofs have been corrected by the authors,
or other paperwork completed.
Not sure I like that.
What's the rush?

253.

My experience as an editor made me question
the value of peer review in its current form.
It was slow, prone to bias and abuse,
and hopeless at detecting fraud.
I was never brave enough
to blind the referees to the authors
and was always at the mercy
of unbending statisticians.

254.
"Firsts" in medical research
used to be much easier to identify than now
when most papers have cohorts of authors
from multiple centres.
I think it is a mistake
to always credit the first or the last author
as the prime mover.

255.
I don't think it was only the relative simplicity
of the amyloid cascade hypothesis
that led to its acceptance,
but also the fact that it was a two-author paper.
Bring back papers
with a maximum of five authors.

U. Language

256.

Be precise.

Orwell[58] warned that "the slovenliness of our language, makes it easier for us to have foolish thoughts".

257.

From an old grouch
to those about to write up research:
Think about what you are saying.
Pay attention to what a word means,
and to the arrangement of words in a sentence.

258.

I have found writing a way of getting a word in,
when nobody has the time or desire,
to listen to my grumbling.
It is a subterfuge for putting the record straight.

---

[58] George Orwell (1903-1950) was an English novelist, essayist, journalist and literary critic.

259.

When talking with patients,
I try to avoid genteelisms and break-teeth words.
Like Bill Shankly[59],
I choose the word greedy rather than avaricious,
and spit or cough rather than expectorate.

260.

My teachers emphasised the value and importance
of writing clearly.
It was as vital in neurology
as being able to communicate well
with patients and colleagues.

261.

The inadequacy of words
makes listening complex.

---

[59] Bill Shankly (1913-1981) was a Scottish footballer and revered
manager of Liverpool Football Club.

262.

Like hearing a new symptom of a disease,
encountering a new word makes life all the richer.

263.

Mark Twain[60] always advised authors
to write mainly short sentences
but to add the occasional carefully crafted longer one too
for variation.
I try to follow that rule
in my own writing.

---

[60] Mark Twain (1835-1910) was an American writer, humourist
and essayist.

V. LITERATURE

264.

Some days I read
to see if I need to change my viewpoint.
Some days I read
to learn new things.
But mostly I read
to travel -
to La Belle Epoque, Aracataca[61],
the Place of Dead Roads[62].

265.

Aleister Crowley[63] used the term 'neuropath'
in the subtitle of his book of poems, *White Stains*.
It is a term which has been lost to medicine,
and might be worthy of resurrection
to describe a certain predisposition to neurological
disorder.

---

[61] Aracataca is the birthplace of Gabriel Garcia Marquez, a
Colombian Nobel Laureate in Literature.
[62] *The Place of Dead Roads* (1983) is the title of the second novel of a
trilogy by William Burroughs.
[63] Aleister Crowley (1875-1947) was an English occultist,
ceremonial magician, poet, painter and mountaineer.

266.

I have been reading memoirs,
including those of Richard Hoggart[64] and Frank
Kermode[65].
Both compare favourably
with the finest autobiographies and nonfiction novels.
Neither seemed motivated by an attempt
to preserve an interesting life for posterity,
but more to explain and educate.

267.

I read *Small is Beautiful*[66] in the seventies.
Other than Marcuse[67], it is the only political book I have
ever read.
It is a defence of the "little men" like Cade and Cotzias,
boutique hospitals like Queen Square,
football clubs like Bury.
Read it if you have time.

---

[64] Richard Hoggart (1918-2014) was an English academic best
remembered for his book *The Uses of Literacy*.

[65] Frank Kermode (1919-2010) was a British literary critic best
known for his book *The Sense of an Ending*.

[66] *Small is Beautiful* (1973) is a book by the German-born, British
economist E.F. Schumacher.

[67] *One-Dimensional Man* (1964) is a critique of capitalism and
advanced industrial society by the philosopher Herbert Marcuse
that became a cult classic in the sixties.

268.

I still advise the students and clinical fellows
to read the Sherlock Holmes canon,
but I have substituted *In Search of Lost Time*,
my other *vade mecum*,
with the superior Rougon-Macquart[68] series.

269.

I was reminded today of Dr Stamford's conjecture
about the Sherlock Holmes metier,
"No man burdens his mind with small matters
unless he has some very good reason for doing so".
We do it to find the cause for symptoms,
Holmes did it to solve mysterious killings.

---

[68] *Les Rougon-Macquart* is the collective title given to a cycle of
twenty novels by the French novelist Émile Zola.

270.

If you have not read *Can Medicine be Cured*[69],
I strongly recommend it.
Seamus has got me to the letter.
Neurology defender of the physical examination,
and of the medical interview,
along with general practice.

271.

A quote I remember,
from *One Dimensional Man*,
and which I think,
is much more relevant to medical teaching now,
than it was in May 1968,
is:
"Who educates the educators,
and where is the proof
they are in possession of "the good"?

---

[69] *Can Medicine be Cured: The Corruption of a Profession* (2019) by
Seamus O'Mahony.

272.

It is well-known that
Joseph Bell[70] was an influence
on Doyle's portrayal of Sherlock Holmes.
But so was Henry Littlejohn[71],
champion of the nascent field of forensic medicine,
and Edinburgh's chief medical officer.

273.

Last week in the Vega[72]
I understood that Lorca[73] had seen,
in his torn-up garden,
the same green winds and roses of blood,
that Cajal[74] had described,
deep in the human brain.

---

[70] Joseph Bell (1837-1911) was an Edinburgh surgeon and one of
Arthur Conan Doyle's tutors.
[71] Henry Littlejohn (1826-1914) was an Edinburgh surgeon, public
health official and forensic scientist.
[72] La Vega is an area of small villages to the west of Granada in
Andalucia.
[73] Federico Garcia Lorca (1898-1936) was an Andalucian poet and
playwright and member of the Generation of '27.
[74] Santiago Ramon y Cajal (1852-1934) was a Spanish
neuroscientist who won the Nobel Prize in Physiology or Medicine.

274.

One of the reasons I read is to remind me
I'm not the only show in town.
I am adapting to the brainhood of the author
and changing colour.

275.

Platforms like GPT-3[75]
can now realistically mimic human creative writing.
Would I enjoy a machine-written extension
to the Sherlock Holmes canon?
I doubt it.
It would all be unblemished,
and stripped of background.

276.

Remember what Hélder Câmara[76] said:
"When I feed the poor,
they call me a saint,
but when I ask why the poor are hungry,
they call me a communist."
Only those who do not seek power,
are qualified to hold it.

---

[75] GPT-3 is a large language model released by OpenAI in 2020.
[76] Hélder Câmara (1909-1999) was a Brazilian Roman Catholic
archbishop, self-identified socialist and liberation theologist.

277.

John Sassall[77] is a good doctor.
He meets the unformulated expectation of the ill
for a sense of fraternity.
Sometimes he fails
because he missed the critical moment to intervene,
or lacked the right words.
But there is about him,
the will of a man trying to recognise.

278.

Sherlock Holmes is the neurologist's alter ego,
but for the neuropsychiatrist,
Inspector Maigret has much to offer.

279.

Sherlock Holmes' method,
like clinical diagnosis,
involved abductive reasoning,
and speculative modelling.
But the difference with real doctoring was,
he knew the perpetrator before he wrote the story,
bearing similarities to a sanitised case report.

---

[77] John Sassall (real name John Eskell) was the protagonist in John
Berger's book *A Fortunate Man,* about general practice.

280.

What I learned from *In Search of Lost Time*,
was that a hundred people,
suffering from the same symptoms,
all will give a different story.
It is up to me to interpret these,
and I cannot do it with a ream of scales,
and tick box questionnaires.

281.

Zola wrote his book on Lourdes[78],
in part because of his interest in the motivation
that leads to the herd instinct,
but also as a description of human suffering,
and the power of kindness and love.

282.

Brian Appleyard[79] wrote about 20 years ago,
that he experienced anomie
as soon as he got off the train at Lime Street[80].
I'm trying to work out why I still get goose bumps
as I go through the turnstile at Manchester Piccadilly.

---

[78] *Lourdes* was the first of Émile Zola's *Three Cities* trilogy published in 1894.

[79] Brian Appleyard is a Manchester journalist born in 1951.

[80] Lime Street is the main railway station of Liverpool.

W. My Writings

283.

My autumnal writing of essays
gives me a satisfaction
because I am at last able to write diagonally
across the page.
It creates in me a sense of holiness.

284.

My book[81], in psychoanalytical jargon,
is referred to as a screen memory.
One can never return to the past,
because it never truly existed,
And the present,
can never be as good as an ideal.
I found I could never go home again.

---

[81] *Brazil that Never Was* (Notting Hill Editions, 2020) by A.J. Lees.

285.

Brainspotting[82] is a demystification
of the study of nervous disease,
and a clarion call
to combine the art of healing
with modern technology.

286.

In *Brainspotting* I tried,
perhaps unsuccessfully,
to leap to the stars,
from a springboard of accurate observation.

287.

I wrote *Mentored by a Madman*
to inspire the young
about the privilege of being a doctor.
The fun as well as the sadness.
And how it is possible to do instructive research,
without a battalion behind you.
See the unseen.

---

[82] *Brainspotting:Adventures in Neurology* (Notting Hill Editions, 2022) by
A.J. Lees.

288.
If your heart aches to return,
to a place you have never been,
If your soul has a sense
of limitless loss,
then read my book,
Brazil that Never Was,
before the snows arrive.

X. COVID Blues

289.

I dream of meetings in Austria,
Finland and Mali.
Although the delegates have removed their masks,
things are no longer the same.
There is a greater distance between us,
and a resignation,
of what has been lost forever.
Friends have turned into holograms.

290.

I have had personal experience,
of my own doctors managing uncertainty better
during lockdown.
I hope that the sadness of COVID
will allow us to release the chains,
tear up the process,
and replace the legal rules with loving care.

291.

My COVID dreams now centre
on aimlessly searching
for unread books
in forbidden libraries,
and on running for empty trains.
No walk in the park.

292.

Since I was grounded,
a recurrent nightmare has been
the rush to catch planes
at anonymous American airports.
Getting stuck in tunnels,
and lost in the neon labyrinth of the terminal,
finally waking in limbo.
Never had these when I was in the skies.

293.

The COVID dreams I remember and write down,
are all about enclosure,
and terrifying entrapment.
I was hoping that I might soar high,
and play in fluffy clouds,
as I did in the days of Asian flu.
But at least I no longer wake,
sweating,
after missing a connecting flight.

294.

We can say with reasonable confidence
that the risk of post-encephalitic Parkinsonism
after COVID
is negligible.
But what we should learn
from the history of encephalitis lethargica,
is the necessity of scrupulous medical follow-up
of all notified COVID survivors.

295.

What has heartened me
is how my colleagues in the current emergency
have by-passed all that stifling red tape
which had blighted our ability
to be good doctors for so long.
They rallied together for society's good,
and put their lives at risk.
They deserve much more than a hand clap.

Y. The Environment

296.

As part of rewilding the lost temperate rain forests of
Britain,
beloved by one of my guides, Richard Spruce[83],
the lichens and mosses must not be overlooked.
Not everything in this world should be commercial,
or for profit.

297.

Deforestation.
Plastic in our organs.
Carbon dioxide emissions.
All horrifying.
But have you considered the pollution of light rubbing out
the stars?
The silence?
The darkness?

---

[83] Richard Spruce (1817-1893) was one of the great Victorian plant
hunters who specialised in bryology and spent 15 years in the
Amazon basin.

Z. Snow

298.

Snow falling silently at night comforts me.
Snow makes me calmer not slower.
Snow makes me want to put my red scarf on.
Snow makes me think.
Snow enhances clinical judgement.

299.

Snow is a cover up that muffles sound.
It reveals and conceals,
it evokes childhood.
Like Carnival,
it eradicates the social order
by cloaking the poverty of the city.

300.

Snowfall is a wonderful canvas
for the writer interested in the kindly murderer
and the superstitious atheist.